Nursing
An Amazing Career

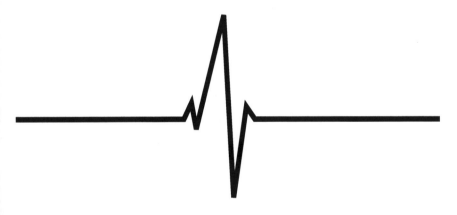

A Book for Potential Nurses, their Patients, and the Curious

Cindy Samborski

NURSING, AN AMAZING CAREER: A Book for Potential Nurses, their Patients, and the Curious

Copyright © 2011 Cindy Samborski

Cover design by Sarah Holroyd
Book design by Sarah Holroyd

NOTICE OF RIGHTS

NOTICE OF LIABILITY

ISBN-13: 978-0983975601

I would like to dedicate this book to my children and my husband for being patient with me throughout my career and helping to make ends meet when I couldn't be there. All my love.

Table of Contents

Preface   1
How it Began   3
Nursing School   7
Patient Education   11
Marrying Education with Clinical Rotations   13
Some Nursing Greats   22
From College to Real Nursing   26
Caring for a Patient on the Medical/Surgical Floor   31
The Oncology Unit   34
Homecare and Telehealth   39
Discharge Planning and Nursing   49
Transition to a Different Type of Nursing   56
Clinical Research Nursing   61
Possible Degrees, Jobs, and Salaries   66
Glossary   72
References   74

Preface

This book is designed to help you decide if you have a real interest in nursing and if you want to pursue it as a career. This book will also help nurses decide how much further they want to go with their nursing career, and what college education could help them achieve their goals. In this book, I explore my path through nursing, including nursing school and the struggles that many nurses encounter each day. I discuss the facts about hospital nursing, homecare nursing, rehabilitation centers, nursing homes, and clinical research in today's healthcare setting. This information will help you understand the many changes, achievements, and advances in the nursing field. In addition, I will discuss the various nursing degrees required for different types of nursing positions.

This book will also provide some insight to patients who want to understand what nurses may deal with throughout their day, and the thought process a nurse uses to make important decisions. You will also begin to understand some of the emotions nurses experience as they treat their patients. Some areas of discussion may be explicit, so be prepared; nursing can be an extremely graphic career. Nursing is full of good times, bad times, and extraordinary times. It's like no other career because its results are directly related to you, your family members, or your loved ones.

Many television shows exist that depict nursing in an unrealistic way. They show beautiful women or men in tight-fitting scrubs.

Physically, nurses are not all thin, healthy-looking beauties. Nurses may struggle with many stressors, and this struggle can become obvious in their appearances. Nurses usually don't fall in love with doctors; their relationship at times can be tense. One of the biggest misconceptions is that nurses have all this freedom to administer life-saving medications. The doctor is the one who makes these decisions and administers these life-saving drugs.

This book encompasses the reality of nursing. It covers the time period from 1989 to the present day, and reveals how research and society also have an impact on nursing and patient care. It introduces you to some nursing greats throughout history and demonstrates how important nursing is to you, me, and our loved ones.

In the 1700s, Florence Nightingale began our crusade, changing the way nurses treated patients. Since that time, nurses have been instrumental in improving treatment of patients, and they continue to change the way patients are cared for in today's age of technology. After reading this book, I hope that you will understand the profession a little better, along with the challenges nurses had to overcome in the past and the obstacles we will face ahead.

The stories I tell in this book are all factual, and I experienced each and every one of them during my 20-year nursing career (and still going strong). I highly recommend nursing as a career and hope this book may tempt you to explore it further. Many nurses have said at one point in time, "I could write a book about everything I have experienced in nursing." Well, this is my book and I hope it motivates and moves you.

Chapter 1
How it Began

In 1988, with two small children and one on the way, I knew I needed to do something to help support them. My marriage wasn't what I had hoped it would be and I felt compelled to act in case I ended up being a single parent. I approached one of my girlfriends about opening up a small business. She agreed and we decided to open a house-cleaning business. Cleaning was something we both excelled at, and it seemed like an easy way to make money and get up and running quickly. So we placed an advertisement in the local Pennysaver and named our company K & C Impeccable Cleaning.

Shortly after the ad was placed, we began receiving phone calls, developed a prominent clientele, and had steady business for three years. We began with cleaning homes and eventually expanded the business to include small stores. Our company brought in steady money, but not enough to live on. On the way home from our cleaning jobs we would stop at the grocery store and usually spend all we'd earned on diapers and groceries.

Cleaning homes benefitted our families and it worked really well for three years. However, this business was something neither of us wanted to expand any further. We grew tired of cleaning other people's homes, just to come home and clean our own. We hired one girl to help us but she didn't perform the way we and our clients expected. It became more of a headache to have someone working for us than to do it all ourselves, because we were perfectionists. We would even walk backwards out of the home, vacuuming away our footsteps as we left the house, so our clients would open the door to a spectacularly clean home.

My partner and I often daydreamed of how one day we would do so well financially that we would be able to hire our own cleaning ladies. One day I did hire someone to clean my home. I was financially stable, but with three children and hockey, softball, volleyball, track, religious instruction, and Tiger Scouts, I didn't have much time to clean my own house. So I called an advertisement in the Pennysaver and had a small cleaning company like ours come to the house. This company had many restrictions as to what they would do and I felt like I had to clean the house before they got there. They didn't wash dishes, they didn't take out the garbage, and they didn't clean baseboards or clean windows. Basically they dusted, vacuumed, and washed the floors with a mop. When I came home after they were finished, I wasn't impressed. It wasn't worth the time or money and no one was as thorough as K & C Impeccable Cleaning! I stopped using them after two cleanings.

Back to my journey into nursing…One morning while my partner and I were cleaning a beautiful home in a lovely suburb, we began brainstorming about other things we could do to bring more money into our households. After we tossed around many ideas, we realized we didn't have enough education to work anywhere and command a good salary. Each of us had only our high school diploma.

We decided to look into colleges and see what they had to offer. Luckily, the local Catholic college was having an open house and we were both able to attend. When we arrived at the open house, I vowed not to go into nursing, because when I was quite young my mother had my sister and I volunteer at a center for developmentally delayed patients. They would act out, and it didn't seem like the nurses had any control over their behavior. This terrified me and I related nursing to this experience. My partner insisted on the nursing program. Ironically, by the time we left the open house I was registered in the nursing program and my partner enrolled in early childhood education. Talking with the nurses at the open house and hearing them explain nursing in a hospital setting calmed my fears. I really wasn't sure if this was the best choice for me, but my drive was supporting my children, and I knew a nursing degree would benefit us. My partner decided she loved working with children and wanted to do something she loved, and becoming educated in that field would suit her best. She went on to open a successful daycare center.

The college offered two nursing programs: a two-year degree program that required students to attend full-time days, and a part-time evening program that completed the degree in three and a half years. I elected to go part-time because I had small children at home. In three and a half years, I would be a Registered Nurse (RN), earn a decent salary, and be able to support my family. I had stars in my eyes, but I had no idea what I was getting into. With this decision, my partner and I promptly stopped cleaning houses and traded our cleaning supplies, buckets, and rags for notebooks and extremely intimidating college books.

Now, you need to remember that back in 1989 home computers weren't as common as they are today. Computer companies were just beginning to market them, and they carried a high price tag, certainly nothing I could afford. In class, we took notes with a pen and paper, and even our computer instructors weren't savvy on computers. During my first computer class, the computers locked up half way through the class and the teacher could not figure out how to rectify the situation. She eventually asked the students if anyone could help get out of the predicament. Eventually, one student was able to figure it out and we were back to work on the computers.

As far as the internet went, it was much different than today. We didn't have options to access it. Our only choice was a dial-up connection. The dial-up connection went through your phone line and you could spend a good hour waiting for your chance to jump on the World Wide Web. Unfortunately, if someone called while you were on the internet, you would immediately lose your internet connection and have to start the process all over again. Can you imagine it? These were my tools in 1989, and with them I was ready to begin my journey.

Chapter 2
Nursing School

To me, learning nursing was like learning a foreign language while living in a foreign country. I didn't have any experience with the medical field except for the short times I was hospitalized to deliver each of my children, and the volunteer work my mother made my sister and I do during the summer at the local hospital. I only worked in the clerical department because at the tender age of 12, I was scared to death of the patients. When I felt a little more comfortable about working in the hospital, I delivered flowers to the patients' rooms, but I made a quick exit once we made eye contact.

My sister, who was a year older than me, worked with patients in the occupational therapy department. She was much more comfortable with patients than I was and really seemed to flourish in that environment. I remember one of her patients was a young guy, about 18. He was a gunshot victim and was paralyzed and had a tracheotomy, a surgical procedure in which an incision is made in the windpipe and a tube is inserted to make an artificial opening to assist with breathing. He was the scariest-looking person I had ever seen, and 18 seemed extremely old. My sister really enjoyed working with him; she didn't see what I saw. Sometimes I talked to him, but would be careful not to look at the whole in his neck. This did help me begin the desensitization process to the medical field, but that quickly wore off once volunteering was over at the end of summer. My sister had real compassion and a special ability to work with patients. She went on to become an RN.

With this minimal experience I was very unsure about patient care, but determined to accomplish my goal of becoming a nurse. I needed to be able to support my family then and in the future. The required nursing curriculum to complete the degree was extremely difficult and potential students had to prove they were capable of success. So prior to my acceptance into the nursing program, I had to take a math and a science class. Unfortunately, they didn't count towards the course requirements, but they showed that I would be a good candidate to handle the nursing curriculum. I aced those classes, but there was no comparison between them and the nursing classes I was about to encounter. Just getting the books alone for nursing classes was overwhelming. I could barely pronounce the words: Anatomy and Physiology, Pharmacology, Microbiology. These books seemed to have millions of pages and be heavier than any book I had ever held. It was frightening, but I knew I was in it for the long haul and had to move forward in order to get through the material.

The nursing program contained the most difficult material I had ever come across in my education to that point, and I knew I needed to develop strategies to learn it. I tried a few different tactics to help me learn and retain the material. For example, after class ended, I would summarize all the information I had learned that day on index cards. I would tape these index cards to the cupboards in my kitchen, where I spent a great deal of my time.

Back then, we didn't have a dishwasher and I spent a lot of time in the kitchen cooking and washing dishes. In addition, I needed to prepare bottles for the baby. For those of you who are new moms, or anyone who has had kids in the last decade, things were much different in the late 80s. For example, to prepare the baby's bottles I had to fill a large metal pot with water. I would then bring the water to a boil and drop the bottles and nipples in one at a time in a meticulous process to sterilize them. I used tongs to get them out, careful not to contaminate them, and then boiled water to mix with the formula. A dozen bottles came out of a batch, and this took a couple of hours. As I prepared bottles I would glance up, read an index card, and repeat it until I'd memorized it.

Another method I used to help me learn the material was to bring my large (and they were large) cassette tape recorders to lectures, record the lectures, and then play the cassettes quietly at night while I slept. My hope was that some of what I was taught would click in my sleeping mind and I would wake up with a new understanding of the nursing process. I do believe that this practice did benefit me because I survived nursing school, but I just can't pinpoint exactly how.

My other strategy was to use study groups. Lots of students formed study groups at school, independent of the professors. I wanted to find a way to learn the material easier or have it driven into my brain in a different format. I could tell some of my classmates were having the same difficulty I was learning and retaining all the material. Nursing students were dropping out of college very quickly. So I asked a couple of my classmates if they wanted to form a study group. They agreed and a group of us got together and decided we would study at my house. I had two small children at home at that time and the majority of the nurses in the study group smoked. I wouldn't allow smoking in my home, so I held the study group in the basement.

A basement during a Buffalo, New York, winter can be quite cold, especially for a bunch of stressed-out nursing students. My basement wasn't finished, just cement blocks and a lot of laundry. I set up a card table, a couple of chairs, and had a stand-up chalk board. We all wore coats, hats, and gloves, and sipped on a 12-pack of beer. This helped relieve a lot of stress, but unfortunately I didn't learn a whole lot.

Eventually the study group ceased, and what I found out about myself after that experience is the most effective way I learn is by teaching a mock nursing class. By speaking the lesson aloud and writing it on a chalkboard I found I retained the information best. I now understand that I am an auditory and visual learner when it comes to learning large amounts of information. If you are a potential nursing student, make sure to try different study techniques. You need to find out what way you learn best. You will find a short exercise at **http://www.acceleratedlearning.com/method/test_launch.html**

that will help you to determine your learning style. There are three basic learning styles: an auditory learner needs to hear what is taught, a visual learner needs to see the lesson, and a tactile learner needs to perform it. You will find one that will work well for you; just don't give up.

Chapter 3
Patient Education

I have to tell you about one story that really made an impression on me. It came from the Obstetrics/Gynecology (OB/GYN) instructor. It really gave me a different perspective on society, education levels, and the role of a nurse. The instructor told us that her day job was working at Planned Parenthood. Planned Parenthood in America is the nation's leading sexual and reproductive health care provider and advocate. They educate young people about birth control and sexually transmitted diseases, and provide counseling and physical exams. This group also serves people with little means of payment and the underinsured. This is the story she told us about one of her patients.

A young girl received a physical exam and was given birth control pills at her request. She was instructed on how to take the pills and the nurse felt confident that the girl understood. She was to return in a few months for a check-up to see how she was doing. About two months later she showed up at the clinic before her scheduled appointment. She had symptoms of nausea, along with a missed menstrual cycle. The clinic gave her a pregnancy test, which came back positive. The young girl was in shock and asked how it was possible that she had become pregnant. She explained to the nurse that she'd waited a month as they'd told her, and that she took the birth control pill every day. The nurse questioned the girl further about her routine. She discovered that the young girl thought she was supposed to insert the pill into her vagina daily to prevent pregnancy. She didn't understand the education she was given, and to her this was the logical way to take the pill to prevent pregnancy.

I was shocked when I heard this story. The lesson learned is that you really don't know what people know or understand. To complicate things further, people may hide what they don't know because they are embarrassed. It is our job, as nurses, to explain, listen, and make sure every patient is taught well and understands what they are taught.

You can run into all types of barriers to educating a patient successfully. Language barriers, cultural barriers, and generational barriers are just a few. And also be aware of illiteracy; it exists everywhere. You would be surprised how many people in today's society are illiterate. People may be raised with little or no education. It's very hard for an illiterate person to share this information with medical staff, or anyone at all. Today, people have to sign multiple forms before they even receive healthcare. People who are illiterate usually have mastered a signature and are happy to sign for you.

As a nurse, you can use subtle devices to check for illiteracy. For example, if there is a pill bottle around, I will ask the patient to read the label. This opens up a comfortable conversation regarding their vision and the nurse can begin to assess their ability to read. Language barriers also hinder a patient's ability to understand.

Patients who cannot understand what a medical professional is trying to teach them can put their health at risk. For example, I have had patients who are prescribed medicine and will just take one pill out of the bottle a day. The medication may be ordered four times a day, and the patient just doesn't understand. To help patients, you have to implement strategies. For a patient who has to take a certain drug once a day, at night only, I will draw a moon on the pill bottle. If they need to take the medication twice a day, I may draw a sun and a moon on the bottle. As a nurse, you must ensure a patient understands what you are teaching them, verify it, and be creative to help them adhere to it.

Chapter 4
Marrying Education with
Clinical Rotations

You've taken classes such as Anatomy and Physiology, Nursing 101, Nursing 102, and Nursing Theory. You are fairly well overloaded mentally, but another component of nursing is added. At this point in your education, the school administration deems you ready to work in hospitals with actual patients, a practice called "clinical rotations." The student nurse works for approximately eight weeks, a few days a week. These rotations are conducted in several different hospitals and include different types of medical floors such as medical/surgical units, oncology units, psychiatric units, children's units, and labor and delivery.

Students spend some time on both the day and evening shifts, and each shift runs a little differently. On the day shift, many doctors see their patients, write new medical orders, and discharge patients. Some patients undergo medical testing within the hospital and are off the floor for a good part of the day. Patients usually bathe in the morning and might have physical or occupational therapy at their bedside or in the therapy department. Patients receive most of their medications, like Intravenous (IV) antibiotics, and various types of treatments, for example, wound care or inhalation therapy.

The evening shift may settle down a bit, but the majority of the duties remain the same. On the evening shift, the nurses continue to care for the patients—administering medication and performing treatments—but less so than during the day shift. Most patients' families visit at this time also. Patients' families usually have many questions for the nurse and the nurse may spend a lot of time with the family. This is discussed in depth in a later chapter.

We were all very excited to begin clinical rotations. We purchased our uniforms from the mandatory, pricey uniform shop. We were required to wear white nursing hats (if you can remember those pristine white hats), white shoes, and white stockings. The group of nursing students arrived in the lobby of the local hospital ready to begin our journey to becoming real nurses.

The day before a clinical rotation, students spend the evening completing prep work at the hospital. The first evening, seven other students, the instructor, and I went up to the medical floor to get our patient assignments, review the records, and devise the next day's plan for when we actually provided care to the patients. The ride up the elevator was very intimidating. I can remember how scared I was. I was still afraid of the patients and was trying to hide it. I was also afraid of not knowing what to do, what to expect, or how to deal with it all.

The nursing instructor led us out of the elevator and down the corridor. It was dinner time and nurses and nursing aides were busy bringing dinner trays into the patients' rooms. The instructor assigned each student a patient. We immediately went behind the nurses' station to the medical chart rack. This gave me a sense of security. I was eager to read the medical records and the diagnosis, although I still didn't know what I was doing. I had a lot of information floating around my brain, but no way to tie it all together. I thought that, in a clinical setting, it would start coming together, but it didn't. Nursing became more overwhelming and confusing. Looking back, I believe this was a normal response.

Once we each had our chart, we gathered in the conference room with the instructor and examined our charts to extract any information we could to get a better understanding of the patient. Even after reading the medical record I could not pull it all together in my mind. I was familiar with some of the terminology, but my confusion continued about exactly what I was supposed to do. On top of that, the staff nurses seemed extremely intimidating. I didn't know if this was intentional on their part, or a feeling I created on my own. However, it did add to my stress level, so I had to ignore it and focus on the task at hand.

After this preparation, the instructor told us to go into our patients' rooms and introduce ourselves. She told us to introduce ourselves and explain to the patient that we would return in the morning to help with their care. I asked the nursing instructor to go with me to see my patient, as I still felt very uncomfortable. As I approached my patient's room, I hovered near the doorway and was afraid to go in, but with my instructor's insistence I finally walked into the room.

The room was dark with a large window revealing dusk. The patient lay in the bed with tubes and monitors with flashing lights connected to her. Her eyes were closed and she lay still. I stared at her for a moment, then turned right around and immediately left the room. I had never seen anything like that in my life. I was in shock. I was afraid and I needed to gather my thoughts and breathe for a minute. My first patient, as a student nurse, was in a coma and not responsive.

With my instructor's urging I reentered the room, and this time I stayed. I stood there for a while staring at her and at all the tubes and machines. I didn't say a word. After a while, my fear began to subside and then I was able to see a woman lying in the bed, a woman who was quite ill. Immediately, my fear returned because I had no idea what to do. To that point my training as a nurse had not provided me with the tools needed to care for this patient. That night when I got home, my fears began to intensify.

The next morning we reconvened at the hospital and went back to the medical floor. We read the medical records again to learn what had happened with our patients during the night. Our duties for the day included assessing the patients physically, taking their vital signs, assisting the patients with bathing, and giving them their medications. Once our plan was in place, we each went to our patient's room. My apprehension began to increase.

When I walked into my patient's room, it was well lit. I looked right at the patient lying in the bed and when she saw me, she said hello. I looked at her again, not recognizing her from the previous night. My patient had woken from her coma during the night. There were still tubes and monitors connected to her but she was conscious, responding, and appearing quite happy. This was the first unbelievable experience I had as a nurse, but I assure you, not the last.

That experience kept me going through the rest of the incredible challenge of nursing school. The amazing human body is so mysterious and captivating, I just needed to learn more. As a nurse, anxiety and fear are two emotions you may experience often, but you will work through them. It's not a fear of the patients, but a fear of the unknown. These are normal feelings you experience while learning to become a nurse. If you decide to go into nursing, you will understand what I am speaking about. These emotions seem to be a part of nursing. They keep you sharp, and when you overcome them, what you learned by doing so will make you a better nurse.

As a nurse, you will need both mental and physical strength, possibly more than you have ever needed before. I assure you this education and experience will change who you are as a person in a positive way. It will change how you perceive and relate to people. It will help you grow intellectually and emotionally. It will provide you with a new appreciation of good health. The outcome is incredible.

Nursing is a very unique process; it's not black and white in any form. A nurse has to understand a patient's medical condition and understand how to treat it. A nurse has to deal with a patient's personality, along with their family (today the definition of a patient includes the family and anyone considered family), the physician, and other medical staff. The nurse is an educator and has to plan outside the immediate hospital surroundings. They plan for what life will be like for the patient when they get home. The nurse has to organize all of these components and administer competent, kind, and compassionate care.

It is said that nursing school does not reflect "real nursing" and I partially agree. How could nursing school ever mimic real patients, their emotions, and real disease processes? The intent of nursing school is to educate you on the human body and disease, and prepare you with the tools you'll need to care for patients. It also familiarizes you with stress and different coping techniques. The human body is unpredictable, and to this day, I'm still learning new things about it. This is why it is impossible for nursing school to capture everything you will encounter in this field.

During clinical rotations, the student nurses have one or two patients at most, in a type of controlled atmosphere. In the real world of nursing, a nurse has many more patients to care for. I'm not going to lie and say hospitals are well staffed with nurses; many times there aren't enough nurses for all of the patients. If you were a patient at one time and reading this book, you may be able to attest to this very fact. However, nurses make do. They become extremely creative and count on the other members of their team to help meet the patient's needs.

Clinical rotations were just the beginning of the challenges I faced in nursing school. Early on, I ran into the problem of a personality clash with a specific clinical instructor. The role of the clinical instructor is to supervise a group of nurses and oversee their practice in the hospital setting, including reviewing nursing assessments. The instructor also oversees such student actions as administering medications, performing injections for the first time, inserting IVs and Foley catheters, and much more. In hindsight, this is an extremely stressful position for a clinical nursing instructor to be in. If a student nurse makes a mistake, the instructor's license could be in jeopardy.

Our first clinical instructor was extremely tough. When we had questions and came to her for help, she would say, "Don't come to me with questions; come to me with the answers." This would have been a good technique, if we'd had any experience at all. One day, she asked me a question in a patient's room in front of a few other students. I didn't know the answer, but another student nurse quickly answered. The instructor then told me (in front of everyone) to quit school, that I would never be a good nurse, and to get out of the profession now. I will never forget that experience and questioned myself and my ability to be a nurse for a long time as a result. I didn't have the confidence or the knowledge to deal with that form of instruction. I dreaded working with that woman for an entire clinical rotation; however, it didn't stop me from pursuing my goal.

The next week I returned to the hospital ready to deal with her once again. When I arrived, there was a new instructor in her place. I asked where the other teacher was and the new instructor said that our previous instructor went skiing, fell, and broke her leg, and she wouldn't be back. She'd told me I'd never be a good nurse, but I've earned two master's degrees and flourish in my nursing career with the same excitement and curiosity I had when I was a student. I wish I could tell my first clinical instructor that today, but I am sure she wouldn't recall her words to me, or really care. One important thing to remember is that you are not shaped by others; you are in complete control of who you will become. If you are a good nurse it's because of you; if you are a bad nurse it's because of you.

Depending on the college you attend, you might have an opportunity to have a clinical rotation on a psychiatric unit. The college I attended did have us complete a rotation at the local psychiatric unit. Before we went to the hospital, we met with our instructor at the college. She talked to us in depth about privacy laws with regard to psychiatric patients. We were instructed never to discuss who we saw or what we did. Today, this practice is not exclusive to psychiatric patients; it's practiced in every healthcare environment and is regulated by the federal government under the Health Insurance Portability and Accountability Act (HIPAA).

When I worked in the psychiatric unit, I was very apprehensive. Today, I can attribute my apprehension to ignorance of what psychiatric illness really was. I did the best job I could based on what I'd learned in class. We completed a six-week rotation at that hospital. The patient I had was so severely depressed that he had become a deaf mute. There wasn't much I could do with a patient like that, except to provide short visits with him to try and establish trust. Unfortunately, it didn't work. He must have seen me as just some young girl trying to communicate with him without a clue as to how to accomplish it. I stayed attentive to him throughout the entire clinical rotation, providing frequent short visits, but he never spoke while I was there.

When you rotate through these different types of venues, you may not always accomplish a good end result because the equation includes an element of unpredictable human behavior. But this element is exactly what makes nursing an interesting field to get in to. The rotations are designed to give you a glimpse at what each medical setting may be like. They also help you decide if any of them is a field in which you may want to specialize. Psychiatric care wasn't a field I was interested in working in; thankfully many nurses love this field.

After the psychiatric rotation, my group of students went to the local children's hospital. Because I had young children at home at the time, I was even more apprehensive to see a sick child than an adult, and a bit emotional about it too. The first day we gathered in the hospital lobby and discussed what we were going to do. We needed to go to our specific floor to get our patient assignments, and briefly review their medical records. We weren't able to visit the patients yet. We then met our instructor in the cafeteria to discuss the care we would need to provide for the next evening.

Once we met the instructor and sat down around her, each and every one of us started to cry. I'm sure it wasn't the first time she'd had an entire group of students break down on their first day of that rotation. It was heartbreaking to see those sick little ones, and we were helpless to cure them. A few of us were young mothers and lucky to have healthy children. The instructor listened to us as we let out our emotions. We eventually pulled ourselves together to discuss the children and how we could best help them.

My first patient was a newborn baby, born to a prominent family that already had one healthy child. There had been no indication that the second child wouldn't be healthy too. Unfortunately, the baby was very ill at birth, and was presumed to be blind. She'd already had major surgery; one of her lungs had been removed and she was recovering. Her parents weren't there the day I was assigned to give her care. I immediately became attached to the baby, and literally couldn't leave her alone while I was there. I stayed with her the entire day to comfort her and make sure her needs were met. I couldn't imagine what it would feel like to be born, undergo immediate surgery, and then lie in a crib alone. I tear up just thinking about that poor little girl, her family, and the devastation that they had to go through. If I heard another baby crying I would put my patient in the baby carrier and bring her with me to go calm that child. These kids are alone because their families have to work and it's heartbreaking. I could never be a pediatric nurse, and I have great esteem for those nurses who are these patients' guardian angels. After clinical rotations you'll get a better feel for where you will want to work after graduation.

My next rotation was OB/GYN, and I was so excited I couldn't wait to start. Finally, I was where I'd dreamed my nursing career would flourish. The rotation wasn't at the children's hospital; it was at the local hospital. The floor was full of mothers getting ready to deliver their babies. It had a cheery, uplifting look about it. The smell of the floor was fresh and clean, not like the other floors in the hospital. I was extremely comfortable and felt perfectly at home. There was a woman about to give birth to twins. She agreed to let a small group of students come observe the deliveries.

A few of us donned scrubs, surgical caps, gowns, masks, and gloves. By the time we got in the room, she had already begun pushing. The atmosphere was electric, and our eyes all filled with tears as the first baby was born. Then a problem occurred; the second baby would not move down into the birth canal. The doctors decided they needed to perform a Cesarean section (C-section) immediately. In a few seconds, the room changed from a birthing room to an operating room, with nurses rushing around getting things ready. The mother appeared worried and elated at the same time, with the birth of her first child. The newborn was whisked away, an anesthesiologist came rushing in, and the surgery began. The second baby was born, and I was in awe. The babies were both healthy, as was the mother. My career goal became at that moment to work in labor and delivery, but labor and delivery is one of the most difficult fields to get in to. After I'd been in the nursing field for a while, my goals changed and I lost interest in labor and delivery and flourished in homecare. This is another benefit to becoming a nurse; you have a wide variety of medical venues to work in. You can continue to grow, learn, and specialize in many different areas.

These were some of my more memorable experiences in clinical rotations. The following are some points to remember if you decide to go to nursing school:

- Many challenges will present themselves and you must persevere to become a nurse.
- You will recognize how the human body coupled with human emotion will impact the disease process, and you will need to treat the patient with these components in mind.
- To be a nurse, you will apply everything you learned in school, along with an entirely different knowledge base which can only be learned through experience.
- It is extremely hard work, both mentally and physically, but has an incredible reward that cannot be found in other occupations.

I highly recommend nursing as a career. The nursing field will continue to grow and require good nurses to take care of the population.

Chapter 5
Some Nursing Greats

I want to provide you with some background on the history of nursing so that you can gain an understanding of how the field has evolved over the years. It includes great accomplishments made by nurses that helped improve the patient's health, procedures for patient care, and patient outcomes.

The nurse has always been a necessity, but lacked social status. Because of maternal instinct, women were considered "born nurses." By the 16th century, the definition of a nurse included "a person, but usually a woman, who waits upon or tends to the sick" (Nursing Power 2011). However, during the 19th century, two more components were added to the definition that stated nursing included "training of those who tend to the sick and carrying out of such duties under direction of a physician" (Nursing Power 2011). The role of the nurse expanded to include care of the sick, infirm, aged, and handicapped, as well as the promotion of general health. The development of nursing depended on two additional ingredients: skill and expertise, and knowledge. The head, heart, and hands have united to become modern-day nursing's foundation (Nursing Power 2011).

There are four inspirational figures who have achieved great accomplishments in the field of nursing. Of all nurses throughout history, Florence Nightingale has become an icon. If it wasn't for her, patient care might be quite different in the world today. Born in Italy in 1820, Florence longed for independence from her parents and a career in a hospital. She trained in a German nursing school and in 1854 she headed to Turkey with a corps of nurses to aid English soldiers wounded in the Crimean War. The conditions of the barracks appalled her. Fleas and rats were everywhere, and the sewers were nearly overflowing, foul air blowing from them through the hospital. Florence decided that better conditions were necessary if the patients were to recover. She established her own laundry with boilers to heat the water and decrease the spread of infection. She had extra kitchens installed in the hospital to ensure that patients had enough healthy food to eat while they recovered. Six months after Florence began making changes in the hospital, the mortality rate had dropped from 42.7% to 2.2%. Florence's methods and successes allowed her to affect military and societal attitudes toward caring for the sick. The military began to understand that the sick needed adequate food, suitable environmental conditions, and proper medical treatment (Cohen 1984).

Can you imagine being 24 years old, wealthy and relatively well educated, with a terrific social future ahead of you, and feeling so strongly about being a nurse that you would give all of that up to serve others? I can't, especially during the 1800s, when the status of women in society was so different as compared to today. Bravely, Florence Nightingale went into deplorable conditions at a hospital and decided that those patients needed better care, healthy nutrition, and sanitary conditions to get well. Her actions improved their health, recovery, and mortality rate. You would think the actions Florence took would be common sense, but they weren't—like many other things we take for granted today. Ideas were developed somewhere by someone for a particular reason.

Another icon who made an impact on the field of nursing was Clara Barton. She is best known for organizing the American Red Cross. Born in 1821, Barton was the "Angel of the Battlefield" during the Civil War in the United States. Once a clerk in the U.S. Patent Office, Barton used her training to organize a supply line for the soldiers on the battlefield. She also went to the battles herself, tending to wounded and dying soldiers. President Lincoln asked her to look for missing soldiers who were captured by the enemy, which helped many families identify those who died in the Andersonville Prison. In 1870, Barton helped the International Red Cross during the Franco-Prussian War, eventually leading to the formation of the American Red Cross in the United States (Nursing Degree Guide 2011).

In addition to Barton and Nightingale, Margaret Sanger was important to the history of nursing. She contributed the design for a diverse organization to benefit society. Born in 1879, she grew up in New York's Lower East Side. Initially, she was a nurse for the underprivileged and began to realize the effects of unplanned pregnancies in those destitute conditions. She left her nursing work in order to promote the use of birth control and give women everywhere the ability to make their own reproductive decisions. At first it was a battle, but eventually her work paid off with the formation of the World Population Conference in 1927. Sanger formed the Planned Parenthood Federation in 1942, which still stands today to educate women about their reproductive health and choices for family planning (Nursing Degree Guide 2011).

Lastly, a nurse who isn't as well known as the other three, but who made a difference to the injured, is Helen Fairchild. She entered the battlefield of World War I in 1917. As one of the 64 nurses from Pennsylvania Hospital Unit Ten, she volunteered to be in the American Expeditionary Force and helped those soldiers who had been wounded in combat. Spending much of her time in a Casualty Clearing Station in Ypres-Passchendaele, Fairchild was one of the nurses expected to cover two thousand beds that filled the small area. This was an unbelievable challenge. From her letters, we learn that Fairchild would stand in mud in order to treat patients and that the pace was chaotic. The base hospitals could offer a measure of backup and rest time, while the casualty clearing stations were expected to treat patients quickly and then send them to a main hospital or back into the field. Fourteen-hour days were not uncommon. Unfortunately, she never made it home to share the stories that she only alluded to in her letters (Nursing Degree Guide 2011).

Today's nurses should also be inspired like these four incredible women. Nurses continue to have the ability to develop new, innovative ways to improve patient care and patient outcomes. Nursing is much more than starting an IV in a patient's arm or administering their medicine. For example, nurses can author, develop, test, and publish nursing research. Nurses can make positive changes in patient care and outcomes. Nurses can identify a problem, research a solution, and devise a plan. They can test the plan through research, and if the results are positive, they can publish them. This is how a nurse can impact practice.

Chapter 6
From College to Real Nursing

Nursing school was a challenge. While I was busy attending school, caring for my children, and studying, it made it difficult to focus on the end result. It was actually one of the toughest things I have ever accomplished. It was obvious that it was a challenge for other students as well. There were originally 50 students enrolled in my class, and it seemed that each week someone dropped out. I remember one girl dropped out because her handwriting was so bad that no one could read it. She tried to improve it, but she could not make it legible. Crazy, right? Especially today, since most healthcare facilities have Electronic Medical Records (EMR) and illegible writing is not an issue. We are forever evolving in the medical community. I can't begin to imagine what it will be like ten years from now. Patients may check in with a lone fingerprint due to the developments in bioinformatics. Doctors everywhere may be able to access your history and medications by turning on their computers. We are only limited by our own minds.

After you have successfully completed nursing school with a B average or better (a C is a failing grade), you have to register for the state boards. In a two-year nursing degree program the college highly advised that students take the Licensed Practical Nurse (LPN) boards first because you need to get experience in taking this type of an exam. Then if you fail the RN boards, you have the LPN license to fall back on and can still actively practice. The nursing exams in school are supposed to mimic the state board exams; they are timed—if I remember correctly, 50 minutes for 50 questions. The questions were complicated, all multiple choice, and usually had two similar answers out of the four choices. You really had to thoroughly understand the question to choose the right answer.

In New York at the time of my exams, the LPN boards consisted of an eight-hour day held at the local convention center. Approximately 200 to 300 nursing students filtered into the convention center. We were immediately relieved of our belongings except for two pencils. The room was extremely large and had high ceilings and rows of tables with two nursing students at each. I was a nervous wreck. The material was broken down into two four-hour sessions. After taking the first half of the exam, my confidence had dwindled. On our short lunch break, the other nursing students talked about right and wrong answers, which made me even more nervous. Take my advice and don't talk about any exam after you take it, especially with people who may have done worse than you.

As we gathered to go back into the room, a group of guys were entering the main door of the convention center. This was the local minor league baseball team in their uniforms. They were young, kind of wild, and you could tell they had just come from a practice or a game. Their entrance completely threw off my exam concentration and for some reason calmed me down and brought me back to reality. I wasn't nervous or tense any more. I went back into the room, sat at my table and finished the exam. Six weeks later, I received the results in the mail and I had passed.

Next I sat for the RN boards. They were two days long in the same environment as the LPN boards. The one major difference between the LPN and RN boards was that there were many more proctors throughout the room. The proctor monitoring my table stood approximately eight feet from where I was sitting. During the exam, he decided to take out his nail clippers and trim his finger nails. The sound echoed in my head like glass cracking. It was a terrible experience, and I was surprised I made it through the day, but I did, and I passed.

Today, nursing candidates go to a testing center in a secure area and take the exam on computers. The students are relieved of all of their belongings and go into a room with multiple other students. The others could be taking any type of exam, all conducted at the same time. The students are each seated at a single desk with a partition on either side so as not to be able to see each other's computers. The students are each given a calculator, pencil, and paper, along with the computer. Each is given a headset to put on to distract them from other sounds in the room. The room has several cameras, one in each corner, and there is a separate room where the staff monitors all the students. Each student logs into the computer and the exam begins. After the student answers a certain number of questions correctly, the computer automatically shuts down. This process of exam-taking is a major improvement over the process I experienced. It no longer takes two full days to complete it, but just one afternoon. The students find out their results in a short time frame. This process allows students to become licensed nurses more quickly, securing their employment.

After I took the exam the old-fashioned way, I was considered a Graduate Nurse (GN), and with a GN status I was allowed to work as a nurse in a hospital setting. The Catholic college that I attended was affiliated with to the Catholic hospital next door. When we graduated, we were sent right over to the human resources office at the hospital. We were immediately given a Math for Medications exam, and if we passed we were hired to work as a GN on a medical floor. Thankfully I was hired immediately and began to work. Your salary was paid as per guidelines for a graduate nurse until you received your passing grade.

GN programs still exist and most hospitals will hire graduate nurses right out of school. There is usually a time lapse that occurs between graduation and finding a testing center that has an available appointment for you to take the exam. Today most nursing employers want a nurse to have at least one year of medical/surgical nursing experience to progress in the field. This is a minimum amount of time to gain a better understanding of the anatomy and physiology of the body, and of the nursing practice. In addition, many management or advancement positions require nurses to have multiple years in medical/surgical nursing or they will not be considered for a higher position. I strongly advise any new nurse to work in medical/surgical nursing for at least three years at the beginning of your career. This way if you want to move into different nursing fields you will already have three years of hospital experience.

In 1991, nursing jobs were scarce. Nursing schools were closing and nurses were saturating the field. Today, it is the opposite; nursing is a stable field to get into. According to the latest projections from the U.S. Bureau of Labor Statistics published in the November 2009 Monthly Labor Review, "more than 581,500 new nursing positions will be created through 2018 (a 22.2% increase), making nursing the nation's top profession in terms of projected job growth" (American Association of Colleges of Nurses 2011). Part of the reason this projection exists is because of the mean age of today's nurses and the number of baby boomers that are beginning to reach their 60s and continue to age. According to data from the latest National Sample Survey of Registered Nurses, nearly 73,000 RNs leave the profession annually due to retirement, child-rearing, returning to school, career change, death, or for other reasons (HRSA 2010). Even though there is a nursing shortage, it is not typical to walk into a day-shift position in a hospital as a new nurse. A nurse today will usually have to start with an evening shift and work their way up to the coveted day shift.

Today, nurse leaders of large hospital systems are joining together to brainstorm and implement new programs that will relieve the nursing shortage. For example, where I practice locally, we have a lack of emergency room nurses, so the nurse leaders have developed and implemented a preceptor/mentor program. This program allows graduate nurses to work with a preceptor/mentor in the emergency room for one year while they take their state board exam and successfully pass it. This new nurse is assigned to a trained preceptor/mentor and after completing the year, a supervisor will decide if the nurse can work independently. The difference with this new program is that this nurse can go from graduate nurse to emergency room nurse in one year without medical/surgical experience. The nurse who enters into this type of specific program must sign a contract indicating that she will work for two years in the same facility, so the company doesn't lose the money they have invested in her training. I think this is really exciting, especially for nurses who want to go straight into the action of an emergency room. A nurse would normally need to work in the hospital, possibly in a specialty unit like a Cardiac Care Unit (CCU) or Intensive Care Unit (ICU), for a number of years before they were able to work in an emergency room. A nurse could fulfill a career goal in a much shorter period of time. If they'd had this type of program back when I was in school I would have signed up immediately. Nurses devised this plan and made it a reality. As a nurse you have the ability to make positive changes and have them implemented, benefiting other nurses and society.

I have seen other changes made during my career in nursing. There have been major reforms made to improve the working conditions. For example, at the time that I began practicing, smoking was just becoming the societal evil that it has evolved into today. The hospital administration had just changed the cafeteria from one large smoking area to separate non-smoking and smoking areas. The ceiling of the cafeteria was completely yellow and nicotine was the prevalent smell. In addition, patients could request a written doctor's order to smoke in their rooms. This illustrates how improvements made in the medical field continue. A simple idea conceived by someone in the medical field may be considered a great idea by the larger society and implemented.

Today our medical campuses are entirely smoke free. This means that patients or employees are not allowed to smoke inside or outside of the hospital. The ashtrays have been removed and the patients are directed to smoke away from the facility. If you do smoke, it is a smart idea to smoke before you come in to work or when your shift ends. Smoking is no longer tolerated in the medical work place. Believe me, I have seen first hand what it does to the lungs and the way it corrupts the beautiful human body.

Chapter 7
Caring for a Patient on the Medical/Surgical Floor

In a hospital, a medical/surgical floor consists of both medical patients and surgical patients. These floors usually have 15 to 20 patients or more, depending on the size of the hospital. They are usually staffed with a variety of RNs, LPNs, and nursing aides. Medical patients may be recovering from an acute or chronic illness. For example, a patient may be admitted with Congestive Heart Failure (CHF), which is when "your heart can't pump enough blood to meet your body's needs. Over time, conditions such as narrowed arteries in your heart (coronary artery disease) or high blood pressure gradually leave your heart too weak or stiff to fill and pump efficiently" (Mayo Clinic 2011). Symptoms may include shortness of breath and retaining extra fluid in their ankles and legs. These patients may need oral or IV diuretics to remove the excess fluid that the heart is unable to remove. The physician treats the patient with the right amount of diuretics to help the patient breathe easier. The patient most likely will need diet modification and close monitoring. These patients may come into the hospital more frequently for these types of treatments and be discharged when they are able to breathe better and are deemed stable by the physician.

In this unit, you may also see cancer patients. It's usually not for chemotherapy but for the side effects of chemotherapy treatment or disease progression (chemotherapy is usually administered on a specialty medical unit). This floor may also include patients with End Stage Renal Disease (ESRD) when they are experiencing complications. Other patients on this floor may need management of their hypertension, diabetes, Lupus, or other disease processes.

Also included in this unit are surgical patients. These patients may include people who are scheduled for hip or knee replacements, patients who may need an exploratory laparoscopy (inserting a small scope in the abdominal area to inspect organs for sites of disease), or patients who may need an appendectomy or their gallbladder removed. The medical/surgical floor can adapt to any type of surgical patient. Patients who undergo cardiac surgery usually recover in a CCU or an ICU.

The nurse on this type of medical/surgical floor starts her day by going into her assigned unit and obtaining the patient report from the nurse who was caring for the patient on the previous shift. For example, nurse A will be responsible for rooms 222 through 228, and each room has two patients. The nurse is responsible for the patients' care on that shift. This includes assessments, bathing, wound care (if needed), administering medication, infusing IV fluids (if necessary), and communicating with the physician and other medical professionals about the patient's condition. There are also various tasks the nurse must complete throughout the day, including recording input and output for some patients (how much they ate or drank and what their output was during a shift), blood work, or other treatments the patient received, along with documenting everything the nurse completed during the day.

This may sound like a lot at first, but it is manageable and becomes a routine. The nurse usually has a nursing aide to help with many of these tasks, along with teamwork from additional staff. Some hospitals have LPNs to assist with some of these duties. Nursing students are usually available to assist on a busy nursing floor at times, too. Nurses have to be extremely flexible and be able to delegate tasks and manage staff. Many patients do very well in hospitals and have great success after a short stay. For example, the nurse may have a patient who needs IV antibiotics and wound care due to an open sore on his leg. After a few days of treatment, the patient is doing well and gets discharged to go home. It is very rewarding to see a patient recover and be released, and this happens most of the time. The story I will tell you next is not typical, but it is about one of my very special patients, Georgia.

She was a young mother and she lay in a private room as a surgical patient. She'd had abdominal surgery due to ovarian cancer. The doctors weren't able to control the cancer no matter what treatment they tried. The surgical site on her abdomen was open and draining and we had to perform frequent dressing changes to try to control the fluid. She had two little girls who would come in and visit once in a while when she was up to it. She stayed on our floor, and to be honest, her case was so sad that I had rather not be assigned to her. As you can imagine, this type of illness caused Georgia terrible pain. We did the best we could to control her pain. The surgeon would come in periodically and do what he could to stitch her stomach closed. Her abdomen continued to leak fluids from her internal organs, and one day I had the realization that she was going to die there with us. Georgia wouldn't be going home to be a mom to her children; her life would end there, in the hospital. Most patients survived and were discharged to go home. I had never had a patient of mine pass away before. You can't imagine the emotions I was feeling, as a young nurse and a young mother. I can still feel the emotion as if it occurred yesterday.

After weeks of caring for Georgia, I came to work the Monday before Easter Sunday and she was gone. I was relieved for her that she didn't have to suffer any longer, but I was sad for her family, her young girls and husband. I knew that we'd given her the best care we could while she was there with us. I knew it would be a long week— the kids were off from school and the holiday was soon approaching.

On Easter Sunday, as I was celebrating the holiday with my children, the phone rang. I answered the phone and the caller simply said, "Is Georgia there?" I was shocked and politely told the caller they had the wrong number. I will never forget that call.

Chapter 8
The Oncology Unit

After spending many nights working 3 to 11 pm and missing my children, I bid on a full-time day job. Even though the job was in the oncology unit, I never thought twice about taking it when it was offered. I'd come from a medical/surgical floor that included orthopedic patients and medical/surgical patients. I thought I could learn what I needed to as on-the-job training in order to care for these patients. In hindsight, I was really young and naïve, both as a person and as a nurse.

There were many different types of patients in oncology. For example, there were patients who were being treated with chemotherapy and patients who had complications due to the side effects of chemotherapy (or their cancer) such that they required medical support to live. The oncology floor wasn't specific to any type of cancer and was an adult patient floor. It was in the oldest part of the hospital, on the fourth floor, and this elevator had a front and a back door. The back door of the elevator opened to the morgue with a special key that we had. This was the only elevator in the hospital that had access to the morgue. So any patient who passed away came through this elevator to the morgue. There were a few private rooms used specifically for hospice patients and about 12 other rooms with two beds in each of them. At night, with less staff than during the day, it sometimes seemed a little spooky.

The nurses who had worked there for years told us stories of things that had occurred. The floor was situated in a T shape, with the nursing station in the middle of the T. There were two rounded mirrors mounted near the ceiling at each corner of the T because when you sat at the nurses' station you couldn't see down either hallway, where the patients' rooms were on either side. The nurses would say that at times during the night, they would hear someone walking up to the nurses' station with loud-sounding footsteps and when they looked in the mirrors no one was there.

They also told a story of a patient who had terminal cancer and was an inpatient for quite a while. This patient fought as hard as he could to beat the cancer and was angry that it would ultimately take his life. After the long battle the patient finally passed away. The nurse on the evening shift said one day she heard the wooden rocking chair rocking back and forth in that patient's room. The nurse knew that there were no patients in that room, so she went to investigate. She thought perhaps a co-worker was taking a break. She said when she walked into the room the chair was rocking back and forth with the patient who had recently passed away sitting in it. The patient smiled at her and then faded away. The nurses said that happened often within that specific room. I think it was rather distasteful to have the morgue on the same floor as the oncology unit. In any event, there are many stories that you will hear, and you have to put them in perspective. This, I believe, was the established nurses trying to put a scare in a new nurse (me), but I really didn't believe their stories. Remember, especially as a new nurse, to keep things in perspective.

The staff on the oncology unit included both mature and young nurses. They all really cared about the patients. There were four doctors, with four completely different styles. One doctor was a young Indian doctor, a striking woman who dressed beautifully, and the patients loved her. One physician was more reserved; his patients seemed to survive longer than the other physicians'. He was truly brilliant and, in a way, mysterious. There was also a young oncologist and a Canadian oncologist who practiced on that floor, but we rarely saw him.

As a nurse, you must learn the physician's style. You learn to work with them, and begin to understand their preferences, as well as their personalities. Working in the nursing field is all about being a part of a healthcare team, especially in an acute care setting. It's critical that everyone works together. The nursing aide, nurse, and doctor work together, and observe and communicate with each other. This is the best way to provide care to the patient.

When I started working in the oncology unit, I began to meet the patients, and trust me, a cancer patient is like no other patient. They are determined. They have a unique perspective on life that you usually don't see in a patient who does not have a serious chronic illness—a perspective that a healthy person can never truly understand. Other patients may be at different stages in their diagnosis like denial or anger. It depends on the patient and each patient is different. You may have two patients with the same type of cancer and they react differently. Cancer is unique to the patient; of these two patients, one might be cured of their cancer with treatment, while the other's identical form of cancer may become metastatic, spreading to other organs within the body.

As nurses, we administer chemotherapy to our patients and work to control the negative side effects. We act as a support system for the patients when their families aren't there. We try to identify where they are mentally with the disease process and help them cope with their feelings. It's really tough sometimes, but it would be much harder to be the patient than it is to be the nurse.

I became more comfortable working in oncology after a while. I worked the 7 am to 3 pm shift and clocked in promptly at 6:45 each morning. The moment I got in, I checked to see which patient rooms I was assigned to. I would quickly stop in each room to make sure everything was all right with my patients before I listened to the morning report from the night nurses, who would tape record everything that happened the evening before. This report prepared us for what we needed to do during the day to meet the patient's needs.

On one particular morning, I went into my first patient's room and discovered that the patient had passed away sometime after the last nurse had checked on him. Most of the patients on the floor had signed Do Not Resuscitate (DNR) waivers, which meant that if they were dying, hospital staff members were not to take extreme measures to resuscitate them. Today, this is covered by a Health Care Proxy statement, which directs the physician as to what measures a patient wants taken in the presence of imminent death. This patient had signed a DNR previously so he peacefully passed away. The next room I went into, the patient had also passed away and was also listed as a DNR. Later that day, we had another patient pass away and this became one of the saddest days in my nursing career.

The fourth patient I had that day was a strong, young man, at least six feet two inches tall, in his 30s, and he had a wife and young children. He had bone cancer, and in my entire career, I don't think I have ever seen a patient suffer as much as he did. At first, he received chemotherapy, but eventually it stopped working and the cancer began to spread throughout his bones. One day he came in for treatment, and immediately became a hospice patient. A hospice patient remains in the hospital to receive comfort care, rather than actual treatment. This includes administering pain medication and providing the 24-hour care these patients require. There are also special counselors that come in and help the patient and their family deal with the grief and other emotions they experience when a loved one is going to succumb to a chronic illness. The ultimate goal is to keep the patient as comfortable as possible.

With the cancer spreading throughout his bones, they became extremely brittle and he was in great pain. No matter how much pain medication we gave him, the pain was uncontrollable; at best, the pain medication took the edge off the pain. Eventually, when he tried to move in bed he would scream out in pain. You could actually hear a bone crack. It was the first time I ever sat at the nursing station and cried. It was one of the saddest things I had ever experienced in my life.

After a while, almost every patient that I admitted I watched die. But we did have some successful patients who beat cancer. Those patients we didn't see any more because they didn't require hospitalizations. One day a 19 year old came in for chemotherapy treatment. He was admitted, but luckily that day he wasn't assigned to me as a patient. I couldn't even look in his room when I walked by. I just couldn't handle the fact that he was so young, and his coming here to be admitted to the hospital made me feel even worse. I wasn't ready to handle that type of patient and I eventually left the oncology setting. I can only hope that he survived.

Oncology nursing is a tough field, but it can be rewarding, helping people to cope with their illness and knowing you offered kindness and support in their final days. In today's oncology environment, many cancers have become curable, many cancers have become manageable, and patients with metastatic disease can survive for years. This is all do to medical research, which I will talk about in a later chapter.

Chapter 9
Homecare and Telehealth

In 1993, I applied for an IV homecare nursing supervisor position. After a couple of years of starting IV lines in patients for chemotherapy, I thought I had become somewhat of an expert in the field. Chemotherapy is tough on a patient's veins and after a while it becomes harder to start IV lines. Today, many chemotherapy patients opt to have ports implanted under their skin; a few types exist. These decrease the amount of needle sticks the patient has to endure for long-term infusions.

I arrived at the interview and found out the company I was interviewing with had two different departments. I thought I was interviewing for the IV homecare nursing supervisor position, but I had made the appointment with the other department for an opening as a community health nurse. During the interview I discovered this mistake and the director asked if I would like to reschedule. I decided to stay for the rest of the interview and hear more about the position. After the three-hour interview, I decided I would like the position and was offered the job.

Homecare was not like anything I had experienced before in nursing. In nursing school, we barely touched on the subject, because there were so many other things that we needed to learn. I also had a two-year degree, and homecare is addressed much more thoroughly in a four-year degree program. In homecare, as a nurse you must use your critical thinking skills. You must be able to act quickly and be prepared for any type of medical problem. Luckily, I had an excellent orientation with an extremely knowledgeable preceptor. Without her insight and education, I might not have survived this very different type of nursing.

The homecare company I worked for wasn't always a homecare agency. It began in the late 1800s as an orphanage and then evolved into housing for homeless women. It was a religious company and the homecare provided was centered on the inner-city population. The majority of homecare rendered was to people who were living at or below the poverty level.

As a nurse, you must remember that when you enter a patient's home, your venue has changed. You are not in a controlled hospital room. When the surroundings change, the nurse must adapt to this change. For example, the nurse does not have easily accessible supplies or another colleague readily available for support. The nurse is alone, with a patient and a piece of paper (a doctor's order). This order tells the nurse what needs to be done, but leaves out how to do it. The nurse must construct the plan. The nursing care plan nursing students learn in college becomes extremely relevant and valuable in homecare. The patient counts on that nurse to know everything medically, and everything that will need to be completed in order to make the patient well again (if that's the patient's goal).

Now, with all these feelings and emotions going on between the nurse and the patient, another critical piece of the puzzle emerges. The nurse must not judge the surroundings she is in, in the patient's home. If the house is messy with six cats running around, the nurse accepts the circumstances and plans her care accordingly. The nurse is not there to judge the patient, but to render care in the patient's home because the physician decided that this was the best place for the patient to receive care. Most patients would rather receive care in their own homes than be hospitalized. The nurse must also put her values aside, as the nurse's values probably won't be the same as the patient's. The nurse really never knows what type of environment she is walking into and must adapt and respect the patient in order to provide the best care possible to facilitate the patient's medical independence.

A typical week for a homecare nurse includes starting your day by going into the office and getting a list of patients that you need to see. These lists are usually organized geographically, with patients in close proximity to one another assigned to the same nurse. Each nurse has a large blue nursing bag weighing about 24 pounds. These bags are filled with medical instruments including thermometers, blood pressure cuffs, dressing supplies, and normal saline, among many other supplies. The nurse may have to see five patients in one day. Each patient may require completely different care. For example, the first patient may have a need for a nurse to provide wound care; the second patient may need an assessment for congestive heart failure; the next patient may need an injection; another patient may need a Foley catheter change and a medication box prefilled.

A homecare nurse has many duties that must be completed throughout the day. The nurse must provide the care, document it, notify the physician if any problems occur, and get the medical record ready for the next homecare visit. The nurse must also track her mileage and complete billing information, along with restocking the nursing bag with any supplies needed. The nurse coordinates care with other disciplines including physical therapy, occupational therapy, nutritional therapy, and social work. These are the standards of homecare; however, many other things can happen that the nurse must attend to. The nurse continuously re-prioritizes her day to meet daily demands. The nurse must also attend staff meetings and educational sessions at the home office. The nurse also has "on call" responsibilities and is required to carry a pager at night and on the weekends. It sounds overwhelming at first, but it's all manageable, especially with a good team. I worked in homecare for 13 years and it was a positive experience. To further help you understand homecare, I will discuss some situations I experienced.

One of the most difficult situations I encountered in homecare was providing care to a young man in his 30s who had ESRD. The treatment required hemodialysis three times a week. Dialysis provides an artificial replacement for kidney function, which fails in renal disease. Patients who receive hemodialysis have a large catheter placed under the skin of their arm. A nurse at a dialysis center accesses the catheter. Blood is moved from the patient through the catheter and then run through a dialyzer. The dialyzer removes waste products from the blood, and then the blood is returned to the patient's body. During dialysis, the patient can become extremely weak due to the entire exchange, which usually happens three days per week over a four-hour period. This is hemodialysis; there are other types of dialysis that can be performed at home through a different type of catheter.

Since his birth, my patient had had a plethora of surgeries to correct other physical problems. He walked with a cane due to his many spinal surgeries; however, he was mainly independent. This young man was also diagnosed with depression. Earlier in his life, he had been instrumental in changing legislation for the disabled. I truly admired him. I was visiting this patient weekly to complete nursing assessments in order to help manage his complicated physical health.

As time went on, I continued my weekly visits with him and he began to feel comfortable with me. He once told me about a girl who he had slowly started to fall in love with. The problem was that this girl was married. From what I understood, he spent a lot of time with her, but it seemed she used him as a sounding board for her personal problems. These problems included her relationships with her husband and child. My patient fell more and more in love with her and wanted to rescue her from this life she was living. One day, she stopped seeing him and stopped talking to him. He was devastated.

Weeks after this, he began to talk about stopping his dialysis treatments. If a patient stops their dialysis treatment, their body is no longer able to get rid of waste products and it poisons itself. Death is imminent. He expressed that he was tired of his life and all the physical suffering he'd endured since birth. As a nurse, I felt he was depressed and called his physician to seek intervention. I really didn't get anywhere with that, so I notified the kidney specialist of his looming decision. Unfortunately, I hit another brick wall. I talked to this young man in depth several times about not giving up, but he just wouldn't listen. His family respected his decision and didn't try to convince him otherwise.

The following week, I called him to set up an appointment time. A family member answered the phone and said he was resting on the couch. They went on to tell me that the hospice nurse was there, and the kindly told me they wouldn't need my assistance any more. I was in shock; he had already begun the process. I immediately asked to speak to the hospice nurse so I could explain my suspicions that my patient's recent depression may be driving this decision. The hospice nurse didn't pay any attention to my pleas.

Four days later, my patient passed away. I received a letter from the family thanking me for everything I'd done for him over the past year. I was crushed, emotionally drained, and didn't know what I could have done to save him. I don't know if my reaction was because it would have been better for me, if he had continued on dialysis. The only thing I did know was that he no longer suffered and he had made this decision on his own. His wishes were respected. I had just wanted to make sure it wasn't a result of clinical depression, but I will never know.

Throughout my nursing career, I have learned that it is not easy to dissociate yourself from patients. Nurses truly want what's best for the patient, but sometimes we just don't know what that may be. You may wonder sometimes if a patient refusing treatment is using it as a surrogate for suicide. My patient clearly wanted to end his life, and by refusing hemodialysis, he knew he could accomplish that very quickly. We all have the right to refuse treatment. However, I made the decision that he wasn't sick enough to want to die. I had no right to do that, as I have no idea how he felt, or how any patient feels. After that experience, I never tell a patient, "I know how you feel," because it simply isn't true.

Nursing teaches you so much about humanity. When you work with people in the most vulnerable position they can be in, you have to use extreme caution. Nurses are a different breed; they look at a patient and see much more than a person. They also have to consider the psychiatric component when they provide care. You cannot truly experience this in school, but must experience it through human interaction.

The homecare company that I worked for created the first HIV homecare team in upstate New York. These nurses were specifically trained to treat the HIV population. In the 1990s, HIV was on the rise. The medications that were prescribed didn't work all that well. Many medications were still in the research phase, and were not given to the general HIV population. During this time, if someone was diagnosed with HIV, the chances of them surviving were slim. Today, patients who are diagnosed with HIV have a more positive outlook. HIV is treatable, although not curable, but a patient can live many years being HIV positive.

My employer was responsible for caring for the largest HIV population in the area. The principal reasons a homecare nurse was needed to treat an HIV patient were education, assessment, and to quickly intervene when acute symptoms arose. These nursing interventions were for newly diagnosed HIV patients who had not yet progressed to AIDS. A large component of the homecare visit was a medication prefill. The nurse would take all the prescription bottles, line them up, and then fill each medication box with the appropriate amount of each pill, at the appropriate time slot. The patients could take 20 to 30 pills a day at different times; it was amazing the patients could still eat with the amount of medication that filled their stomachs.

Patients who had progressed to AIDS usually presented with much more severe symptoms, including massive weight loss, the inability to fight infection, and terrible mouth sores, among the many other things they could develop. Many of our AIDS patients had pneumonia and needed special breathing treatments. Because HIV/AIDS care was funded by the government the doctor could order a nursing aide to help the patient in their own home 24 hours a day. The nurse would have a large care plan to manage with the additional services the patient required.

One of my first HIV patients lived in a very nice suburban area. The patient went into the hospital with multiple health problems and was discharged home with a new diagnosis. I called his local physician and we discussed the hospitalization. I advised the doctor that his patient was diagnosed with HIV. The physician replied that it was impossible because HIV hadn't spread in the suburbs yet. Surprisingly, this was the doctor's actual response. This is how new the diagnosis was early in the 1990s.

I never minded working with HIV patients because, to me, it was just another unfortunate disease. If you maintained universal precautions (avoiding contact with patients' bodily fluids by wearing medical gloves, goggles, and face shields), you were safe when rendering care. One particular nurse wouldn't work with HIV patients because she said she didn't know enough about the disease. This was frowned upon by the rest of us, so she quickly learned the disease process and ended up joining the HIV team of nurses.

During my homecare career, I eventually became a liaison nurse. This is a nurse who assesses new patients for homecare, educates the community and physicians about homecare, and carries out multiple other duties. While working as a liaison nurse, I was asked to assess patients for admission into our homecare program or into the housing unit for the HIV population. This housing unit was a large, old home with approximately 30 rooms. It included a big, beautiful kitchen, sitting areas, and plants. The first floor contained about ten rooms for the sickest patients. The second floor housed sick patients, but they were more independent. The top floor contained small apartments with patients who were able to maintain independence with some assistance. This house included specialty staff and counselors, and was manned by our HIV nurses.

One day I received a call to assess a patient who lived in an apartment in the inner city. I talked mainly with the patient's brother and set up the assessment appointment through him. As a homecare nurse, you need to be aware that you may be providing care to patients in high-risk cities that could be dangerous. Therefore, my company contracted with a security agency and, if a nurse felt the need, we could have a security guard accompany us to a patient's home. Something made me feel uneasy about the entire meeting and my instinct told me to bring a security guard. I called our security agency and they sent our regular guard. He was a small man (smaller than me) with white hair and a limp because he was in need of a hip replacement. Usually, having a security guard present would diffuse a potentially bad situation. We met at the office and I drove us to the patient's home. His brother insisted on being present during the appointment and that sent up a red flag. He alluded to the fact that he wanted to make sure his brother was fine with this appointment. The way he conveyed this to me made me feel uneasy.

We arrived at the home and the patient seemed a bit angry. His brother was telling him to calm down. The patient was an African American man; about six feet three inches tall, with a muscular build. His eyes were intense when he looked at me, like his anger was building. In my mind, I was setting up an escape plan in case I needed to get out of his small apartment with only one door. Although I was very uncomfortable, as an assessor nurse, I needed to have the patient sign an HIV release of information.

I sat in a chair with a small table separating us. His brother stayed standing and my security guard also sat down. I explained to the patient what I needed him to do, and I placed the consent form on the table and handed him my pen. All of a sudden, the patient picked up the pen and stabbed the consent form on to the wooden table and ripped the page with a back and forth scraping motion. I immediately got up and bolted for the door. The patient screamed behind me, "I am going to kill the white b*tch!" and ran after me. Thankfully, his brother blocked him and held the door closed after I'd gotten out. I could hear pounding on the door as the patient tried to get out. I ran as fast as a bullet down the street to my car without stopping. I didn't even think about where the security guard was, until he appeared a few minutes later. He asked me why I'd run, with some anger in his voice. I explained to him that I'd run so I could live. He then told me that he had a concealed gun, even though it was not allowed. I am really thankful that I ran; I certainly wouldn't have wanted to witness the guard pointing a gun at a mentally disturbed patient. I followed up with his brother right after that and told him that when the patient got some psychiatric help, I would come back to see him. I never heard from them again.

Next, I would like to introduce you to Telehealth, if you're not already familiar with it. Telehealth is making its way throughout the country as a means of monitoring patients and providing communication between patients and healthcare workers. A large number of people are linked to the internet and expect more options from healthcare providers. Telehealth and the internet may be the best way to meet the needs of patients who otherwise may not receive care at all.

Telehealth has become a growing need of patients for a few reasons. Computer-literate baby boomers will expect access to healthcare systems using multiple forms of technology. In addition, older adults without prior computer skills are now the fastest growing cohort of internet users and use the World Wide Web mostly to access healthcare information (Merrill 2009). In addition, the isolated and underserved populations can now be reached and services can be provided using text and video modes of communication across the internet. Healthcare services delivered to patients in their homes include patient assessment, post-acute care monitoring, and the provision of internet-based health and mental health interventions (Marziali, Dergal, and McCleary 2005).

Most Telehealth systems include a basic set-up package that many agencies buy including blood pressure cuffs, scale, thermometer, and oxygen saturation measurement tools (Jackson 2006). Patients are instructed on the proper use of each device which are all attached to the Telehealth unit. If a patient is unable to demonstrate proper use they cannot be a candidate for Telehealth.

The Telehealth and e-Health technologies are of enormous assistance to patients and healthcare providers. A comprehensible assessment of a patient must be conducted to judge if the patient is a candidate for the Telehealth program, and both the patient and the provider must agree on Telehealth use. The healthcare organization is solely responsible for the security of the patient's personal information communicated back and forth from the patient's home to the medical office.

Most large homecare companies have a division of Telehealth. Both homecare and Telehealth nursing positions usually require a bachelor's degree. This type of job is for the more independent type of nurse, who can think quickly on her feet and communicate well. In homecare, you can be put in critical situations with a very short time to respond. You must be self directed and possess excellent critical thinking skills. In Telehealth, the nurse needs to be able to communicate well with patients and have sharp skills to assess when a patient could be getting into trouble medically. I recommend both of these positions for the experienced nurse.

Chapter 10
Discharge Planning and Nursing

After I had been a nurse for 15 years, I applied for and accepted a position in a large hospital setting within the Discharge Planning Department. My role was to identify patients who would need homecare, sub-acute rehab, medical rehab, or long-term placement. The goal of the Discharge Planning Department is to ensure patients receive a safe discharge and can continue to recover at home, or in the appropriate facility. As an assessor nurse, I assessed patients, determined their needs, and made recommendations on the next level of care the patient required.

These types of nursing jobs are critical to a patient's safe discharge and recovery. Upon a patient's admission to the hospital, certain built-in triggers will alert the discharge planning department that a patient may need the help of an RN upon discharge. These triggers can include a patient over the age of 75, a patient needing wound care, a patient with a chronic disease, a patient who is hospitalized frequently, or anything else that puts them at risk for a poor recovery. A floor nurse providing care to a patient can also order discharge planning, along with the patient's physician, if they identify specific needs that are not being met and will hinder the patient's recovery.

Before I talk about the job description, I need to get you in the right frame of mind. This is how a nurse must be thinking to assess and treat patients while making discharge planning decisions. The patient's treatment extends beyond the patient. The nurse must view the patient and family as one unit. You may be thinking, "How can you treat the patient and the family?" If you think about this for a minute, the patient's family plays a significant role in the patient's care and recovery, whether the patient is in the hospital, the doctor's office, or in homecare.

For example, I had an 86-year-old patient who lived alone. Her daughter visited her three times a week and brought her meals and groceries, cleaned her home, and reminded her to take her medications. When I saw my patient and her daughter interact with each other, I noticed her daughter put her mother off a bit, and it was apparent she was showing signs of stress about having to care for her mother. In addition to her treatment plan, the patient also needed to receive an injection daily. When I mentioned the injection to her daughter, she verbalized how much time she already spent caring for her mother, and that she was always away from her own family and responsibilities.

This scenario is very important to the nurse planning the patient's care. The nurse may ask if there is anyone else who helps out at home. The nurse must also be sensitive to the daughter's feelings and needs. Caregiver stress is a reality in today's society. An important factor that nurses should be aware of is overworking the caregiver. If the daughter burns out, the patient may end up with a lack of care, become hospitalized, or even placed in a nursing home. We can offer solutions to deal with these types of situations. But we must be aware of them first. Many times discharge planners will call family meetings to identify key members of the family willing to help. The nurse may contact a homecare company to educate patients and family members on self injections. The nurse can also provide information about assistance from other groups that are available to help the patient. Many groups exist to provide support, even support groups for caregivers. This scenario only touches on what can occur with other family members. The impact can be positive or negative on the recovery of a patient. I hope this gives you a better understanding of treating the patient and the family.

An example of a routine referral for a hospital discharge planner is a patient who was hospitalized with a new diagnosis of insulin-dependent diabetes. The patient does not drive, does not have a family, and can ambulate with a cane. The discharge planner reviews the patient's information when the patient is admitted to the hospital. Next, the discharge planner discusses the details of the patient's home situation and her level of understanding of her new diagnosis. The discharge planner may then order homecare for the patient, along with a visit from the hospital nutritionist. This type of homecare is usually provided by a Certified Home Healthcare Agency (CHHA). This type of homecare is usually short-term, with a defined plan of care. The homecare nurse delivers a glucometer, insulin syringes, and other necessary supplies to the patient's hospital room. The nurse then instructs the patient about how to use her blood sugar testing kit and how to administer insulin injections.

The patient is then ready to be discharged from the hospital and is sent home with her supplies and a lot of knowledge. The homecare nurse reports to the patient's house the next morning to see if she is able to use her glucometer and self inject the insulin. When the nurse arrives, she notices that the patient is presenting with some confusion and is also complaining of weakness. The nurse tests the patient's blood and the result on the glucometer reads 56 (this is low, confusion and weakness are signs of hypoglycemia).The nurse quickly goes to the patient's refrigerator to get her some orange juice or something sweet to raise her blood sugar. The patient drinks it and five minutes later the patient's confusion resolves. The nurse takes another blood glucose reading and the result is 98, now within normal limits for a glucose reading.

While in her fridge, the nurse notices that the patient has minimal food. The nurse must investigate why the patient has so little food in her home. In doing so, she discovers that while the patient was hospitalized, she wasn't able to reach the person who normally shops for her. They discuss her options, and the patient decides she wants help with creating meals and learning her new diet. The nurse discusses with the patient the Meals on Wheels program and the patient agrees to receive these services. The nurse makes a referral for the patient to have Meals on Wheels. The nurse identifies the need for further instruction on nutrition, the use of her glucometer, insulin injections, and hypoglycemia, and then notifies the doctor of what occurred.

Because the patient is homebound (not able to leave without a taxing effort), her insurance company will pay for homecare services. The homecare nurse visits the patient the next two days and then three days the following week. By this time, the patient is receiving Meals on Wheels and she has learned to use her glucometer and self inject insulin. The patient now understands the importance of nutrition and her diabetes. The nurse notifies the physician and deems the patient independent in her own care and closes the homecare case. This would be a typical hospital discharge homecare patient. The discharge planning begins when the patient is admitted to the hospital and ends when the patient is independent. Each nurse, no matter what job title she has, plays an import role in the discharge planning process.

In New York State, a long-term home healthcare program exists. This program is also referred to as a nursing home without walls. It is a Medicaid program designed to provide homecare services that can equal up to 75% of the cost of having a patient in a nursing home. This program works well because the patient can have an RN managing their homecare weekly. This program has proved to decrease hospital admissions, infection, and other acute illnesses. Services that are available include physical therapy, occupational therapy, speech therapy, nursing aide services, Meals on Wheels, and a life line. A life line is a button that a patient wears around their neck or wrist that, when pushed, allows the patient to obtain help from a healthcare provider. The nurse has two goals for the patient's recovery. One is to manage the developed plan of care for the patient in their home and all additional therapy services rendered. The other, and the most important, is to identify signs and symptoms that would indicate the patient is becoming acutely ill. The physician can then intervene early on, preventing the patient from experiencing worsening symptoms, and preventing hospitalization. If hospitalization is needed, it can be handled in an expedited manner, again to control worsening symptoms of disease.

There are other discharge plans from the hospital, based on patients' needs. You may know a friend or relative who had knee replacement surgery and then entered a rehab center for physical therapy. When a patient has surgery such as a knee or hip replacement, they will usually go to a sub-acute rehab center a day or two after surgery. Many hospitals have inpatient sub-acute rehab centers; however, many off-site sub-acute rehab centers exist. These rehab centers try to attract patients to come and tour their facility before surgery and reserve an inpatient room. Many health insurance plans will reimburse rehab centers for this type of care, which promotes a faster and healthier recovery.

A patient can be admitted to a sub-acute rehab center for other reasons besides surgery. A patient who is hospitalized can become de-conditioned quickly, which means the patient has become extremely weak and needs daily physical and occupational therapy to recover their strength. Rhabdomyolysis, which is the rapid breakdown of skeletal muscle, can occur when a patient falls in their home and remains in the same position for a long period of time. These patients are extremely weak, but after physical therapy, they usually recover.

A nurse who works in a sub-acute rehab center assists the patient with bathing, administers medications (which may include IVs), and adheres to the rehab regimen. The nurse continues with patient education, assessments, pain evaluations, and wound care if needed. The nurse communicates with the therapists and the physician to design a discharge plan once the patient becomes independent. The patient is seen by the specific physician provided by the rehab unit, possibly twice a week. The patient could still require homecare after this discharge if their needs haven't fully been met.

Another type of rehab is medical rehab, which is a unit within the hospital for patients with more complicated illnesses who require intense rehabilitation. The patient may have had cardiac surgery and needs physical, occupational, and nutritional therapy daily, and close monitoring by the physician. The physician must see the patient daily. If a patient requires this type of care, the insurance company will reimburse the hospital at the same rate as an inpatient hospitalization (or close to it). Patients who complete this program can be discharged from the medical rehab unit home, or be discharged to a sub-acute rehab unit, depending on what meets the patient's needs the best.

In both types of rehabilitation units, the physicians, therapists, and the discharge planning nurse hold weekly meetings, which are designed to identify the patient's progress, establish new goals, and facilitate the best discharge planning for the patient.

Assisted living is another option for discharge planning. Assisted living facilities allow people to move into a home environment. These are usually private pay facilities and the environment is clean and modern. These are for patients who are not ready for a nursing home, but should not live alone. These facilities have staff 24 hours a day but the patients are not fully dependent on the staff. The patients usually need assistance with bathing, meal preparation, and some activities of daily living. However, they still can do many things for themselves.

Another option is a long-term care facility, where residents receive 24-hour care (often called a nursing home). This option is for when a patient can no longer be cared for at home either because the care requires the skills of a nurse around the clock, or there is not enough family support to provide the care needed. Patients live in nursing homes because they are no longer safe at their own homes.

Lately, private pay facilities have been popping up in many suburban locations. These are usually dubbed "life care facilities" and require a large amount of money to move in ($200,000+) and a monthly rent payment. Many of these facilities return the money upon the resident's death to the patient's beneficiaries. Life care facilities usually impose an age requirement (over 65). The resident moves into a luxury apartment which offers many elite amenities.

There may be a chef on staff, a formal dining room, and usually a café. The facility may have an indoor gym and pool with water aerobics and trainers. There may be a billiard room, along with a piano bar and library. It might also have a workshop with the most modern wood-working tools. It could have all types of classes offered for the residents, along with different types of clubs they can get involved with. The life care facility usually has all of the same rehab capabilities as inpatient facilities. So if a resident needs to go to sub-acute rehab, they go within the life care facility. If they need assisted living or long-term care they can also receive this level of care within the facility. A resident moves in because they want security in the latter part of their life, and this is exactly what they receive in this facility, if they can afford the hefty price tag.

Chapter 11
Transition to a Different Type of Nursing

After working in homecare for about ten years I decided I wanted to do something different as a nurse. The position I held at the time, although a good job, took a toll on me mentally and physically at times. I wanted to learn more and progress more in my career. I decided to go back to school and get a bachelor's degree. The program I entered was one evening a week and took 15 months. With three children, this seemed to be the most manageable route to accomplishing my goals. The bachelor's degree was called a bachelor's of science in management. I completed the program and moved on to my next position, discharge planning. Unfortunately what I discovered about the degree was that most nursing positions required a bachelor's of nursing, not management. This was another roadblock I faced. However, I did secure the discharge planning position, partially because I had earned a bachelor's degree.

About a year into my new position, I required a hysterectomy. This meant eight weeks off of work, in the summer, initially with many physical restrictions. By the second week of recovery I was bored out of my mind and entered the master's program at the University of Phoenix, completing the Master's of Science in Nursing (MSN) and Master's of Health Administration (MHA) programs entirely on-line. For those who want to know how attending college on-line is, I will tell you. It's a challenge; you don't have teachers teaching the courses, you have facilitators. Facilitators evaluate your work to assess whether or not you are meeting the course objectives. You are given a number of assignments and questions and you post the answers to an on-line environment. Other students, along with the facilitator, comment on your responses. You write approximately 100 papers and a practicum (similar to a thesis), and become quite proficient in writing. You are self taught and you must research everything until you find the right answer. I feel I have learned more being self taught. Graduate school changed me, by helping me to develop who I was on a personal level. I believe each degree made me view life differently by presenting different views of life to me. Education expands your thought process, personality, and outlook, and changes your perception of external situations and circumstances. You become more open minded, you question more, and you understand so much more. It's a very positive experience that promotes professional and emotional growth.

I was heavily involved in my education, working, and raising my children, and one day during this time period my entire life changed. Nurses don't usually go around thinking that what they see happening to their patients could never happen to themselves or their family. Nurses usually hope that their families don't have to experience what the patients we care for have experienced. But sometimes we do.

At the tail end of my homecare position, our family received terrible news. My sister, who was in her early 40s, was diagnosed with colon cancer. She had been bleeding rectally for about a year and never told any of us even though my other sister and I are nurses and my brother is a doctor. My sister was beautiful, a model for a while, and received healthcare through a clinic. In this clinic there were many new, young physicians who rotated through the practice, learning as they practiced. My sister told the doctor seeing her that she had been bleeding rectally and he never examined her. He told her it was probably hemorrhoids, and she went with that. I don't know why he didn't examine her. Was he too embarrassed to perform a rectal exam on a young woman? We don't know and we never will. Finally when she went to her gynecologist and told her she was bleeding rectally, the doctor immediately performed a rectal exam and found a tumor the size of a grapefruit. My sister was diagnosed with stage IV colon cancer. I tell this story because I want people who have this problem to be checked out thoroughly as colon cancer is curable.

After being diagnosed, she went to who we thought was the best medical oncologist in the area, but unfortunately we discovered through his treatment of her that he wasn't. When you have stage IV cancer, as she did, CT scans are normally performed on your body about every 12 weeks. These scans reveal to the physician if the cancer is spreading. Along with CT scans, a blood sample is usually drawn to check Carcinoembryonic Antigen (CEA) counts. CEA counts, also called tumor markers, can rise in the presence of tumor growth. My sister called to get the results, and the CT scans were normal. She went in monthly for her blood draws to check if the tumor markers had changed. If the tumor markers were normal, the office would not call her.

About a month after she had her blood drawn she called to make an appointment with the oncologist. The secretary went to schedule her appointment and told her she needed to get in there soon, and asked her if anyone had called her about her tumor markers shooting up the previous month. My sister was shocked; not only did her markers go up, but no one called her and when she did find out it was from a secretary. During this time we had thought my sister was in remission, but she wasn't; her cancer was growing and she was receiving no treatment at all. This was the last thing he ever did wrong to her.

She was treated by that oncologist for about nine months and then she went to our local cancer institute, which is one of the top ten cancer institutes in the nation. Treatment for stage IV cancer seemed almost hopeless. But we went to the cancer institute and she found some hope. She met a wonderful, brilliant young physician who used cutting-edge treatments. And when treatment seemed to be futile, she was offered and accepted a position in clinical research trials. She lived for about four years, receiving chemotherapy and radiation during this time, but the cancer was stronger than she was and eventually spread to her lungs. One evening she was admitted to the institute and we all went to see her and she told us she was going home in the morning. She passed away at noon the next day.

While she went through her treatments at the institute she'd always tell me that I should work there. At that time I could not even consider it; the institute was not a happy place for me, and emotionally I knew I wouldn't be able to do it. It took me a while but about three years after she passed away, I did. I applied and interviewed to work in cancer research. I wanted to help find the cure. As fate would have it, I ended up working directly under her doctor whom I so admired for many reasons. Today, I work there as the research educator, teaching others to safely and adequately perform clinical research. The next chapter will explain in depth what clinical research is.

After my sister passed away on March 18, 2005, my family was devastated, as you can imagine. My other sister came up with a great idea to keep our sister's memory alive: Lisa's Legacy. She thought we should educate the public and fund cancer research. The last thing my sister did before she passed away was to enter clinical research even though she knew the research drug she was taking might not help her, but could possibly someday help her son, her family, or others who were stricken with colon cancer. The drug that she actually went on was Avastin, which is now Food and Drug Administration (FDA) approved and used in the treatment of colon cancer.

On Mother's Day of the year she died, we presented my mother with a card that announced the first annual 5k run, raising money and awareness for colon cancer. Over the last five years we have donated over $100,000 to the institute through our fundraising, and Lisa's Legacy remains alive and well. Today it is an established endowment for colon cancer research at the institute. Lisa would have done the same thing for any of us. It's been very hard; we all miss her so much. But this endowment keeps her alive in our hearts; not only for us, but for other patients, family members, and medical staff who knew her and knew of her fight, and knew what she wanted to leave for the others fighting colon cancer.

Chapter 12
Clinical Research Nursing

The main goal of nursing is to provide high-quality patient care. Clinical practice without research is practice based on tradition without validation. Research plays an important role in the nursing profession because it validates each action taken. There are many types of research that exist. For example, clinical and basic research can be used to focus on disease prevention, quality of life, or health disparities. Nursing research develops knowledge to "build the scientific foundation for clinical practice, prevent disease and disability, manage and eliminate symptoms caused by illness, and enhance end-of-life and palliative care" (National Institute of Nursing Research 2011).

This type of research also involves nurses developing their own techniques through research and then applying them to the medical field. For example, Florence Nightingale introduced sanitation as a nursing practice and the results were extreme. Florence documented everything she observed; she noted how the changes she made in her practice positively or negatively impacted the patient's health. She began with baseline statistics on the patients as she first encountered them. She documented their environments, their appearances, their illnesses, and their treatments. She then analyzed all the data she had gathered and thought about what would need to change to promote the patients' health and healing. She documented these strategies, and implemented each one. She observed the changes that occurred in her patients' health and fine tuned her strategies to gain further improvements. She documented a decrease in the rate of infection in her patients and was able to share her new strategies with the medical community and prove how effective they were. This is nursing research.

Nursing research is extremely important to the progression all of nursing practice in today's medical environment, along with the potential benefits it can have for patients. Nursing research can be conducted in a wide variety of venues, including health care facilities, people's homes, classrooms, and hospitals, to name a few. Nurses can develop this research and make it possible to improve patient care.

Another type of research role a nurse can perform is as a clinical research nurse. This is different from the nursing research described above because it involves a nurse implementing another's research. This research can include a new medicine, a new type of medical intervention, or gaining insight from patients on their feelings or emotions during a specific illness. Research in this form is extremely important to the advancement of medicine. Testing new drugs on patients is crucial to this process. Research nurses assist the physician in finding qualified candidates for this type of research. Research nurses explain to the patients what the purpose of the study is and what will happen to them if they agree to be a part of the study. Research nurses closely monitor these patients for any problems that may occur while they participate in the research study. They are also charged with making sure the study is conducted the way it was intended so that any findings or conclusions drawn are valid.

The research nurse inputs everything that has occurred with the patient into a database. The nurse may also need to draw blood samples, schedule specific testing, or follow up as needed for the study. This information is then given to a statistician to compile so that physicians and scientists will have the necessary facts to either prove or disprove the research. Such research can support and validate new techniques and new drugs to treat patients.

Through my experience as a nursing researcher and as a clinical research coordinator, I learned that all research is highly regulated to protect the research participants and to ensure the integrity of the research. Many years ago, the protection of the participants was not a top priority for researchers. Some researchers would enroll a vulnerable population in their research, such as prisoners or orphaned children. These physicians and researchers didn't see a problem with this practice. They thought it was a good way to test research. Other physicians, scientists, and the larger community became involved and this practice ceased; research became highly regulated by the federal government under the FDA.

The research institute where I work requires all employees to become well versed in both the Belmont Report and the Declaration of Helsinki. The Belmont Report attempts to summarize the basic ethical principles that researchers should follow while conducting their research. The Report is a statement of "basic ethical principles and guidelines that should assist in resolving the ethical problems that surround the conduct of research with human subjects" (National Institutes of Health 2011). The Declaration of Helsinki states that "research with humans should be based on the results from laboratory and animal experimentation, research protocols should be reviewed by an independent committee prior to initiation, informed consent from research participants is necessary, and research should be conducted by medically/scientifically qualified individuals" (National Institutes of Health 2011a).

The impact that research has had on society is great. For example, without research, you wouldn't have the ability to take ibuprofen when you have a headache or antacid when you feel some burning in your throat. All drugs must go through extensive research, must be proven effective, and must meet the approval of the FDA in order to be sold on the market. Successful research and results take years to accomplish. For example, it may take up to ten years to get a new drug on the shelf for consumers to buy.

In order to conduct medical research, a researcher or investigator must first design and write a research proposal about why they believe this new drug will be effective. Included in the research proposal are statistics that illustrate their thought process and their prediction of a promising outcome for patients. This proposal is usually prepared by physicians or scientists. A research study is a huge undertaking and must be designed and scrutinized by many different people to confirm its relevance and safety. Research begins with studying statistics, analyzing comparisons, or even by observing treatment of a diseased mouse in a lab.

I recently visited the lab at my facility and saw multiple cages of the cutest little white mice with big pink eyes and long pink tails. Because I don't work in that department, I asked the technician to explain the process. The mice are bred without immune systems so that they cannot fight off disease on their own. To prepare a mouse for this study, a small area on its side is prepped with over-the-counter hair removal cream such as some women use on their legs. Once the area is free of hair, cells are injected from a cancer tumor, and a tumor quickly begins to grow.

After the scientist confirms the mouse has cancer, it is given the drug or treatment designated by the research study. The researchers watch the mouse for a period of time to see if the drug will kill the cancer cells. After a large amount of proof of a positive outcome is gathered, along with other data, the study can be moved into the approval process to be used on humans. It then becomes a Phase One study (there are many different phases of research) to test the dose and safety in humans. The people who enter a Phase One study have exhausted all other treatment options with no positive results. This is usually the only chance they have left.

Any type of research proposal must go through many different layers of departments at a research facility and also before an Internal Review Board (IRB) before it can be implemented. The IRB is made up of doctors, scientists, community leaders, and lay people to keep it objective. After the research study is submitted to the IRB, they may come back and request changes that they feel are necessary. The researcher must make the changes to the proposal and resubmit it for approval. After the IRB approves the proposal, it can be assigned a research coordinator and implemented. The research nurse then helps the physician locate patients who may be interested in participating in the study.

There are many different types of research. We may have a research study that adds a non-chemotherapy agent to the standard of care the patient would already receive. For example, a patient is receiving chemotherapy weekly. The research study adds a vitamin C tablet one hour before the chemotherapy to see if the chemotherapy works better with this additional medication. Another research study may ask a patient to simply fill out surveys while they are receiving chemotherapy to see how it affects their self esteem. Many types of research exist—all designed to help physicians find better cures and treatments while maintaining a patient's quality of life. The nurse is a critical element in achieving quality research.

Chapter 12
Possible Degrees, Jobs, and Salaries

According to the Bureau of Labor Statistics (BLS), nurses make up the largest segment of the workforce within the clinical healthcare industry in the U.S. at over 2.5 million (Santiago 2011). If you want to become a nurse, you need to determine which nursing degree is required for the career you want. Currently, there are five different types of degrees that are offered to nursing students: associate's degree, bachelor's degree, masters of science degree, and two types of doctorate degrees. By the year 2013 the Nurse Practitioner Program will require a doctorate degree.

An Associate's Degree in Nursing (ADN) is a two-year degree that is obtained from a community college or vocational school. An ADN is the minimum requirement to become an RN. However, many employers now require a bachelor's degree for a large number of RN positions (Santiago 2011a).

A Bachelor's of Science in Nursing (BSN) is required for many, but not all, nursing careers. A BSN, like most bachelor's degrees, is typically a four-year degree from a university or college. It combines classroom learning with hands-on training in the form of clinical rotations, which allows students to obtain first-hand experience working with patients in a clinical setting. The bachelor's degree has a larger focus on community healthcare than the two-year degree (Santiago 2011a). When looking for a college, make sure you are enrolling in an accredited nursing program.

In order to obtain your MSN, you must have a BSN or a bachelor's degree in a related field. However, if you opt for one of the combined bachelor's/master's programs, you will avoid this requirement. Furthermore, an MSN is required to become an Advanced Practice Nurse (APN or APRN). APNs have more clinical authority and autonomy, and typically earn more than non-APNs, because they specialize. In addition, other master's nursing programs may include a focus on certain medical specialties or types of nursing, such as a focus on forensic nursing or a clinical nurse specialist track (Santiago 2011a).

A specialized master's degree is also required to become a mid-level provider, such as a Nurse Practitioner (NP) or a Certified Registered Nurse Anesthetist (CRNA). Master's degrees typically involve one to two years of additional coursework beyond the degree program itself that you can obtain while employed as a nurse. Sometimes your employer will help pay for your master's degree in nursing if you commit to working for them for a certain number of years. An MSN must also be completed from an accredited nursing program (Santiago 2011a).

The highest degree you can earn in nursing is a doctorate level degree. You must first have a master's degree before completing the doctorate degree in nursing and become what some refer to as a "Doctorate Nurse." There are two types of doctorates in nursing: a Doctor of Nursing Practice (DNP), which focuses on the clinical aspects of nursing, and a Doctor of Nursing Science (DNSc, also DSN or DNS). The DNSc is the more common choice for those who wish to become professors in nursing programs or researchers. Finally, before becoming licensed and practicing as a nurse, you must pass the National Council Licensure Examination for Registered Nurses (NCLEX-RN) or for Practical Nurses (NCLEX-PN) (Santiago 2011a).

The future goal of nurses, along with the medical professional community, is to eliminate two-year programs and have all potential nurses complete a four-year degree program. So if you are serious about nursing as your career, I recommend completing a four-year degree to obtain a BSN. This program is well rounded and will teach nurses many different nursing styles.

After graduating from a 15-month accelerated bachelor's of science management program, I realized that the nursing world doesn't really acknowledge this program. Unfortunately that meant I wasn't able to get any job in nursing that required a bachelor's degree. When I went back to school to receive my MSN, I had to complete a bridge program, which involved additional nursing classes at a bachelor's level, before the administration accepted me into the MSN program. The bachelor's of management turned out to be a large cost, with no real use to me as it related to nursing. Luckily today, many schools offer accelerated RN to BSN programs, which I highly recommend.

There are many different types of nurses, and several different ways to obtain nursing careers. Just about anywhere doctors work, nurses do too, including hospitals, doctor's offices, clinics, hospices, emergency rooms, intensive care units, government agencies, attorney's offices, and corporations. In fact, nurses also work in other areas where physicians typically do not, such as home healthcare and schools. According to the BLS, over half of all nurses in the U.S. work in hospitals (Nursing Jobs Help 2011).

The average annual compensation for a nurse is between $43,000 and $63,000, with the top 10% of nurses earning over $75,000 (Santiago 2011). The top three nursing fields, based on annual salary and industry demand, are CRNA, NP, and Clinical Nurse Specialist (CNS) (Santiago 2011b). CRNAs basically work as an extension of anesthesiologists, delivering anesthesia during surgery, with an average annual salary of $100,000 or more (Santiago 2011b). CRNAs have one of the highest salaries among the nursing field. An NP is a mid-level provider who provides patient care under the supervision of a licensed physician. NPs are qualified and authorized to conduct patient exams and some minor procedures and tests. A CNS is an advanced practice nurse who also assists with specialized research, education, advocacy, and sometimes management. In addition to being RNs, CNSs also hold MSNs and they have completed the additional CNS certification for their area of expertise. The average salary for a CNS position is between $70,000 and $80,000 (Santiago 2011b).

Another option is working as an LPN. This career requires a General Equivalency Diploma (GED) or high school diploma to gain admittance into the field. The length of the LPN educational program is about a year and can be taken at a local Board of Cooperative Educational Services (BOCES) or a community college. The potential nurse will have classroom education and clinical rotations at local hospitals. At the end of the course, the nurse must take and pass the LPN Boards for their specific state.

An LPN can work in a hospital, a doctor's office, a nursing home, or some homecare nursing agencies. The nurse's duties will exclude some medical practices, as per company guidelines and state law. For example, the LPN will not be able to push IV medications or start IV lines. Pursuing an education as an LPN is a great start into the medical field and can allow you to begin working quickly after the year is over. Many colleges offer LPN to RN programs and many employers are now paying for their LPNs to earn their RN degrees.

An RN is a nurse who has completed either a diploma in nursing, a BSN, or an ADN, and who has also passed the nursing certification exam for RNs. Newly graduated RNs can make between $40,000 and $60,000, depending on their location or willingness to relocate. In 2010, the median income for all RNs in the U.S. was over $55,000 (Santiago 2011a).

If you are an LPN and want to complete the RN program, please check with your current employer and local union, along with the college, to see what they can offer you to complete the program. Also, your goals may change, so be prepared because you might want a bachelor's degree and end up going back to school.

APNs have fulfilled the general RN requirements, and then continued on to study at the master's level or beyond. APNs typically focus these advanced studies in a particular medical specialty in which they obtain a deeper level of knowledge and experience, whether it be oncology, anesthesiology, pediatrics, etc. APNs are some of the highest paid nurses, and include CRNAs, which are the most advanced of all nurses, CNSs, and NPs.

Nursing is one of the most in-demand job skills in America. As you can see, there are different degrees required for different positions. Nursing has become one of the better paying occupations in America over the last several years. In addition to money, opportunity, and job security, there are lots of other benefits to becoming a nurse. There's a severe shortage of qualified nurses to fill all the available positions, and that shortage is only going to get worse. Presently, the shortage is somewhere between 100,000 and 150,000 nurses nationwide (Nursing Jobs Help 2011). The health care industry is not able to fill all its open nursing jobs now, and more nurses are needed every year in most cities. Hospitals and medical offices compete vigorously to hire nurses, and wages, benefit packages, and hiring bonuses are increasing all the time. Furthermore, because of the coming wave of baby boomers reaching retirement age, people living far longer than ever before, and millions of people immigrating to America every year, it's not hard to see why nurses will continue to be in such demand.

I hope you have enjoyed this small glimpse into the nursing profession. If you're a patient reading this book, I hope you have a better understanding of the nurse's perspective. If you're someone who decides to pursue nursing as a career, this information should help guide you to a degree program that will best suit you. Once you obtain a nursing license, your job opportunities are abundant. The field of nursing continues to redefine itself, branch out, and evolve. You can work in a wide variety of venues including hospitals, attorney's offices, for the FDA, in research, or in a school, just to name a few. You are in control of where you take your career. I assure you, you will never be bored, as nursing provides endless challenges.

A nursing career is a journey that develops your strength, intelligence, kindness, patience, and focus. It keeps you grounded in reality and appreciative of life. It makes you sensitive to society and its needs. It exercises your skills of hope and caution. The rewards are endless when you are dealing with humanity. I highly recommend the field.

Glossary

ADN—Associate's Degree in Nursing

APN—Advanced Practice Nurse

APRN—Advanced Practice Nurse

BLS—Bureau of Labor Statistics

BOCES—Board of Cooperative Educational Services

BSN—Bachelor's Degree in Nursing

C-section—Cesarean section

CEA—Carcinoembryonic Antigen

CHF—Congestive Heart Failure

CHHA—Certified Home Healthcare Agency

CNS—Clinical Nurse Specialist

CRNA—Certified Registered Nurse Anesthetist

DNP—Doctor of Nursing Practice

DNR—Do Not Resuscitate

DNS—Doctor of Nursing Science

DNSc—Doctor of Nursing Science

DSN—Doctor of Nursing Science

EMR—Electronic Medical Records

ESRD—End Stage Renal Disease

FDA—Food and Drug Administration

GED—General Equivalency Diploma

GN—Graduate Nurse

HIPAA—Health Insurance Portability and Accountability Act

ICU—Intensive Care Unit

IRB—Internal Review Board

IV—Intravenous line

LPN—Licensed Practical Nurse

MHA—Master's of Health Administration

MSN—Master's of Science Degree in Nursing

NCLEX-PN— National Council Licensure Examination for Practical
   Nurses

NCLEX-RN—National Council Licensure Examination for
   Registered Nurses

NP—Nurse Practitioner

OB/GYN—Obstetrics/Gynecology

RN—Registered Nurse

References

American Association of Colleges of Nurses. 2011. "Nursing Shortage." Accessed May 4. http://www.aacn.nche.edu/Media/FactSheets/NursingShortage.htm.

Cohen, I. Bernard. 1984. "Florence Nightingale." *Scientific American* 250(3):127-138.

Health Resources and Services Administration (HRSA). 2010. "The Registered Nurse Population: Initial Findings from the 2008 National Sample Survey of Registered Nurses." Accessed March 4. http://bhpr.hrsa.gov/healthworkforce/rnsurveys/rnsurveyinitial2008.pdf.

Jackson, Sara. 2006. "Telehealth bears fruit." *Success in Home Care* July/August.

Marziali, E., J. Dergal, and L. McCleary. 2005. "A systematic review of practice standards and research ethics in technology-based home health care intervention programs for older Adults." *Journal of Aging and Health* 17(6).

Mayo Clinic. 2011. "Congestive Heart Failure." Accessed February 12. http://www.mayoclinic.com/health/heart-failure/DS00061.

Merrill, John. 2009. "Continuing Care Retirement Communities." Accessed December 8. http://www.docstoc.com/docs/37437002/ElderNet-Continuing-Care-Retirement- Communities.

National Institute of Nursing Research. 2011. "What is Nursing Research?" Accessed June 1. http://www.ninr.nih.gov/.

National Institutes of Health. 2011. "The Belmont Report: Ethical Principles and Guidelines for the protection of human subjects of research." Accessed April 22. http://ohsr.od.nih.gov/guidelines/belmont.html.

National Institutes of Health. 2011a. "World Medical Association Declaration of Helsinki: Ethical Principles for Medical Research Involving Human Subjects." Accessed April 22. http://ohsr.od.nih.gov/guidelines/helsinki.html.

Nursing Degree Guide. 2011. "Famous Nurses Throughout History." Accessed May 4. http://www.nursingdegreeguide.org/.

Nursing Jobs Help. 2011. "Nursing Careers." Accessed June 10. http://www.nursingjobshelp.com/nurse_career.htm.

Nursing Power. 2011. "Origin of Nursing." Accessed May 10. http://www.nursingpower.net/nursing/origen.html.

Santiago, Andrea. 2011. "Nursing Career Profile—Overview of Nursing Careers." Accessed June 10. http://healthcareers.about.com/od/healthcareerprofiles/p/Nursing_Career.htm.

Santiago, Andrea. 2011a. "Types of Nursing Degrees." Accessed June 10. http://healthcareers.about.com/od/educationtraining/p/Types-Of-Nursing-Degrees.htm.

Santiago, Andrea. 2011b. "Top 3 Nursing Careers: Highest Paying Nursing Careers." Accessed June 10. http://healthcareers.about.com/od/compensationinformation/p/TopNursesSalary.htm.

Made in the USA
Charleston, SC
27 October 2011